THE 5:2

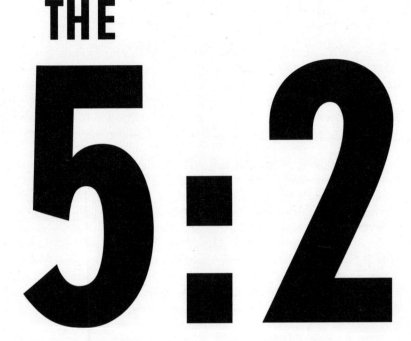

FAST DIET
FOR BEGINNERS

The Complete Book for Intermittent Fasting with Easy Recipes and Weight Loss Plans

Rockridge Press

CONTENTS

INTRODUCTION

Fasting, in various forms, has been practiced for centuries. Many people practice fasting as part of their religion or in preparation for some type of spiritual experience. Others use fasting as a means of periodically cleansing their bodies of built-up wastes and toxins. Some people claim that periodic, short fasts sharpen their focus and clear their minds.

Fasting has also been used by many people as a way to lose weight and body fat. This reason for fasting has become extremely popular in the last few years. This is partly due to many books and websites that have come about promoting fasting as a weight-loss strategy.

There are as many types of fasting diets as there are reasons for fasting. Some are meant to be long-term weight-management plans and others are intended as short-term solutions. While there are healthy versions of intermittent fasting plans, many are far from nutritionally sound. These diets often recommend fasting for too long, invite dieters to eat whatever they like on non-fasting days, or lack guidelines that will help the follower make good nutritional decisions in the future.

The 5:2 Fast Diet is an intermittent fasting plan that encourages followers to eat plenty of whole, nutritious foods on both fasting and non-fasting days. It's not only a healthier alternative to some popular fasting plans, but is also much easier (and more pleasurable) to stick with than some of the more extreme intermittent fasting diets.

Losing weight and body fat is about more than looking good temporarily; it's about *feeling* good, learning to eat in a healthy and sustainable way, and improving your overall health and quality of life.

That's the mission of the 5:2 Fast Diet.

(1)

WHAT IS INTERMITTENT FASTING?

Intermittent fasting is not a starvation diet. On the other hand, it's also not a way to eat a steady diet of junk food and get away with it.

Intermittent fasting is a planned schedule of eating that allows you to eat a normal, healthy diet most of the time, and then requires you to spend a short period of time consuming far less food. There are some intermittent fasting plans that divide fasting and non-fasting periods into mere hours, such as eight hours of eating followed by twelve or sixteen hours of fasting. More commonly, intermittent fasts are divided by days of the week. On the 5:2 Fast Diet, you eat a "normal" diet for five days of the week, interspersed by two days of fasting.

Although the research on intermittent fasting is still in the beginning stages, there is sufficient evidence that eating in this way can help to shed fat, regulate some of the hormones associated with obesity and hunger, and even improve overall cholesterol levels. (We'll discuss the many possible benefits in greater depth in Chapter 5.)

Because intermittent fasting can have a beneficial effect on the hormones that stimulate fat storage and hunger, it can be a very useful strategy for losing weight and shedding body fat. It can also be a very good way for people who don't otherwise follow a healthy diet to break addictions to foods that are unhealthy and learn to make healthier food choices overall.

On the 5:2 Fast Diet, you eat a healthy diet that is close or equal to your daily caloric requirements for five out of seven days. On the two fasting days, women consume 500 calories per day while men consume 600 calories. Because you'll still be eating during the fasting days, this method of intermittent fasting does not generally lead to overeating on non-fasting days, which can be an unwelcome side effect of other fasting plans.

Who Should and Should *Not* Try Intermittent Fasting?

Most people can safely follow the 5:2 Fast Diet; however, you should consult your doctor before beginning the diet, since it is not recommended for some people.

People Who Are Not Good Candidates for the 5:2 Fast Diet

In particular, women who are pregnant or nursing should not attempt intermittent fasting. The calorie guidelines for the fasting days are simply too low. However, once you have had your baby and/or have finished nursing, intermittent fasting can help you get your pre-pregnancy body back.

People with type 2 diabetes should not undertake this diet. Although some evidence shows that it may correct imbalances of or insensitivity to insulin, once type 2 diabetes has been diagnosed, fasting is not advised.

People with a history of eating disorders should not go on a fasting diet. If you feel that you may have an eating disorder or that you're at risk of developing one, it is not recommended that you try the 5:2 Fast Diet.

Children and adolescents should not go on the 5:2 Fast Diet. Please consult a pediatrician or nutritionist if you are seeking a weight-loss plan for anyone under eighteen years of age.

People Who Are Well-Suited for the 5:2 Fast Diet

The 5:2 Fast Diet can be a great plan for anyone who is otherwise healthy but would like to lose weight and shed body fat. However, the format of the diet can make it especially beneficial to some specific groups of people.

People who currently eat an unhealthy diet: People who eat a good deal of fast food, processed foods, and sugar can benefit from the 5:2 Fast Diet's nutritionally balanced approach. The focus of both fasting and non-fasting days is on whole foods: primarily lean meats, fresh fruits and vegetables, low-fat dairy, and whole grains. Many people find that after eating this type of diet for a few weeks, they are better able to appreciate healthier whole foods and have a better understanding of what makes a well-rounded diet.

People who are addicted to sugary foods or empty calories: Many people become addicted to sugary foods, high-carbohydrate processed snacks, and empty calorie beverages such as sodas and blended coffee drinks, which have lots of calories and little to no nutrition. For some of these people, the 5:2 Fast Diet can have the added benefit of helping them break those addictions. This is not only because of the focus on whole foods but also because of the calorie restrictions on fasting days. When you only have 500 to 600 calories to use in a day, it's hard to justify spending half of it on one cola. After a week or two of living without those foods, many people report that the cravings and withdrawal symptoms subside.

People who need an especially simple plan: Some people just naturally do better when steps and choices are very limited. A diet with too many variations and choices or that requires too much planning and decision-making are often hard for such people to maintain. The 5:2 Fast Diet is simple, straightforward, and mapped out step by step. Because of calorie limitations, the fasting day meal plans are extremely simple, and recipes often have just a few ingredients.

How the 5:2 Fast Diet Fits into a Long-Term Plan

Although the 5:2 Fast Diet can be used as a short-term solution for weight loss, it can also fit into your overall nutritional lifestyle.

As we discussed in the previous section, the 5:2 Fast Diet can be a good way for some people to learn the guidelines for making healthy food choices and to begin appreciating healthier whole foods. This can have a very positive impact on your diet long-term.

You may also find it beneficial to occasionally follow the 5:2 Fast Diet if you feel that old habits are creeping back into your life. This can be helpful if you have been eating poorly for a short time, such as during the holidays or while on vacation. Even if you haven't gained weight, you may feel the need to "clean out" your body and start fresh.

If you choose, you can certainly adopt the 5:2 Fast Diet as a permanent way of eating. If you reach your goal weight but want to be able to indulge a bit more on non-fasting days or if you just like the way you feel on the 5:2 Fast Diet, it's perfectly fine to stay on the diet indefinitely. If you are at your target weight, you may want to increase your calorie allowance on non-fasting days so that you don't continue to lose weight.

If your work or lifestyle requires a lot of eating out, or if your diet is not always under your control because of social commitments or scheduling, staying on the 5:2 Fast Diet long-term can help you to balance out your overall weekly calorie intake. Fasting two days per week can counter a less-than-ideal diet the rest of the week, but this is not an invitation to intentionally gorge on unhealthy foods and then "make up for it" later.

Regardless of whether you choose to follow the diet temporarily, occasionally, or permanently, the 5:2 Fast Diet can help you to lose weight, shed body fat, feel more energetic, and gain control over your eating habits.

THE ONE-MONTH 5:2 FAST DIET
WEIGHT-LOSS PLAN

The guidelines for the 5:2 Fast Diet are intentionally simple and straight-forward. Diets that are too complicated or too time-consuming are very hard to follow long enough to see results.

The first thing you will need to do is calculate your daily caloric needs. On your non-fasting days, you will either be eating a diet equal to your caloric needs (for weight maintenance) or 500 calories less than your caloric needs (for weight loss of one pound per week).

There are several good caloric calculators online that you can use to determine your daily caloric needs. You'll enter your gender, height, weight, age, and activity levels. Be sure that the calculator you use does allow you to calculate for regular exercise, a strenuous job, or anything else that will demand more calories each day. Don't use a BMR (basal metabolic rate) calculator, as your basal metabolic rate only accounts for the calories you need to keep your body functioning.

There are several good caloric calculators available, including at:

- FreeDieting.com
- MayoClinic.com
- ACEFitness.org

Once you have calculated your regular daily caloric needs, you can determine your maximum non-fasting intake. For example, if you are an average woman, your regular daily caloric need is approximately 1,800 calories. If you are trying to lose weight, your maximum non-fasting daily calories would be 1,300. If you're a male with a regular daily caloric need of 2,200 calories and you just want to maintain your weight, you would eat 2,200 calories each non-fasting day.

On the two fasting days, regardless of your regular daily calorie calculation, women are limited to 500 calories per day and men to 600 calories.

You'll have five non-fasting days along with two non-consecutive fasting days. Your fasting days don't have to be on the weekend; they can be any two days you think will be easiest for you to fast.

For the entire one-month plan, you'll observe five non-fasting days and two fasting days in each seven-day period. The fasting days should be non-consecutive. Sticking to a two-day-in-a-row fast can be difficult unless you have experience in fasting. It could also set you up for failure.

Fasting Days

In Chapter 6, you'll find several delicious recipes for meals that are 250 calories or less. While you can use these on non-fasting days, they were created to make it easy for you to plan your daily eating on fasting days. On fasting days, if you have calories left over, you can choose items from the list of snacks provided at the end of Chapter 6.

Although we provide a one-month fasting plan for you, you can also feel free to mix and match recipes and meal suggestions once you get acclimated to the 5:2 Fast Diet.

Non-Fasting Days

In Chapter 8, 9 and 10 you'll find many delicious recipes based on nutritious whole foods. The focus of your non-fasting days should be fresh fruits and vegetables, fish and seafood, lean meats, nuts and seeds, legumes, whole grains, and healthy fats such as avocados, olive oil, and coconut oil.

You can use the recipes in Chapter 8, 9 and 10 to create your meal plans for non-fasting days throughout the month and you can also use recipes of your own. Just be sure to get a wide variety of fruits and vegetables each day and try to vary your protein sources, rather than getting stuck in a chicken breast rut.

It's important that you eat plenty of delicious foods that you really enjoy on non-fasting days, as this will help you stay motivated on fasting days. It's a lot easier to fast if you know that you'll be back to enjoying some of your favorite foods in a matter of hours.

What You Can and Cannot Eat on the 5:2 Fast Diet

The following are few hard-and-fast rules about what you can and cannot eat on the 5:2 Fast Diet.

Allowed Foods:

- Fresh vegetables
- Fresh fruits
- Lean meats and poultry
- Fish and seafood
- Low-fat dairy
- Whole grains
- Legumes (such as beans and lentils)
- Nuts and seeds
- Healthy fats (such as avocados, olive oil, coconut oil, flaxseed oil, and nuts)
- Limited amounts of sugar, honey, and sweet treats (see Chapter 11 for low-cal dessert and treat options)

Foods Not Allowed:

- Fast foods
- Deep-fried foods
- Artificial sweeteners

A Note about Carbohydrates and Sugar

There are no specific rules about how many grams of carbohydrates you may consume on the 5:2 Fast Diet, but your non-fasting days should be fairly low-carb. This just means that you should get more carbohydrates from vegetables than from fruit, and more from fruit than from grains. Sweets and desserts are allowed on non-fasting days, but they should be once-a-day or every-other-day treats.

One of the purposes (and benefits) of intermittent fasting is the regulation of insulin levels and insulin sensitivity. If you're taking in a lot of simple carbohydrates such as sugar, bread, and cereals on your non-fasting days, you'll be more likely to have blood sugar spikes, which create a surplus of insulin in your bloodstream. Switching back and forth between high-carb days and low-carb days (such as your fasting days) can make you more susceptible to developing insulin resistance. Insulin resistance, or metabolic syndrome, can lead to excess abdominal fat, heart disease, and type 2 diabetes.

A Note about Beverages and Hydration

It is very important that you maintain proper hydration for good health. This is especially important on the 5:2 Fast Diet, as staying hydrated will help you to feel less hungry, particularly on fasting days.

You must drink a minimum of 64 fluid ounces of water per day! Some people find this easier if they freeze several water bottles to carry with them throughout the day. You can also pack several bottles in an insulated cooler bag to take with you to work.

On fasting days, beverages are limited to:

- Water
- Unsweetened black coffee
- Unsweetened hot tea (without milk)
- Unsweetened iced tea

You'll find that the 5:2 Fast Diet is quite easy to adjust to after just a couple of weeks, perhaps even less. It's best to stick with the menu plans we've provided for the fasting days for at least the first month, since the calories have already been calculated and the menus have been created to ensure that you get a good balance of proteins, carbohydrates, nutrients, and healthy fats.

Once your body has gotten used to this healthier way of eating and you have a good idea of proper portioning and the types of foods you should eat, you can feel free to create your own meal plans and use outside recipes for fasting days.

10 TIPS FOR MOTIVATION AND SUCCESS

1. Try to avoid temptation sabotage.

One thing that can sideline your efforts on fasting days is the temptation of other foods in your fridge and pantry. If you're fairly susceptible to visual temptation when it comes to food, you may want to shop every few days for groceries rather than stocking up once every week or two. Another thing that can help if you have family members or roommates who will not be following the 5:2 Fast Diet is to ask them to tuck away any particularly tempting forbidden foods.

2. Organize your fridge to make fasting days easier.

Try to assign your fasting day ingredients to one shelf of the refrigerator. This can help you train your eyes (and your mind) that only those foods are available to you on fasting days. Eventually, you may find that your eyes don't wander all over the fridge, looking at foods you cannot eat.

3. Remember that socializing doesn't have to involve food.

Eating can be a great part of your social life. Sharing good food or a few drinks with friends and family is a part of our culture. However, there are lots of other things you can do to have fun on fasting days that won't involve eating. Focusing on those activities will help keep your mind off of food but ensure that you don't have to become a hermit when you're fasting. Invite some friends out for a game of tennis, take in an art show, spend a day at the beach, or sign up for a dance class with a pal.

4. If you're a trigger eater, outwit the triggers.

Many of us have certain triggers, aside from mealtimes or hunger, that signal us to eat. Break time at work may send us automatically to the vending machine. Watching TV may be equated with snack time. Maybe you tend to pick at the leftovers on your children's plates as you clear the dishes. Spend the week before your diet making note of all the times you snack, and then create a plan to deal with those triggers while dieting. Make break time at work the opportunity to get in a ten-minute walk. Have other family members clear the plates after dinner. Do needlework, cut coupons, do some stretching, or chew gum when you're watching TV.

5. Set up a reward system.

The best way to reach a major goal is to set several smaller ones and then celebrate them as they're achieved. For every pair of fasting days completed or every pound lost, give yourself a little treat. It could be a manicure, a new book, a night at the movies with your spouse, or just an hour to yourself at the park.

6. Get your friends and family on your team.

Let your friends and family know that you're going on a fasting diet and give them an idea of the guidelines. Even if they don't support the diet, they can still support you by telling you how great you look and not showing up at your home with a dozen donuts.

7. Buddy up.

One of the most motivating things you can have when starting any diet is someone who's doing it with you. Find a coworker, friend, or family member who would like to try the 5:2 Fast Diet so that you can support and encourage each other.

8. Take it one day at a time.

Sometimes just thinking about being on a diet for an entire month can overwhelm you. Try to focus on one day at a time. Adopt this attitude: "I don't have to stick to my diet tomorrow, I just have to stick to it today." Of course, you're going to repeat that *every* day!

9. Learn to tell the difference between hunger and other feelings.

Most of us do a lot of mindless eating. We eat because we're angry, we eat because we're bored, or we eat because we're tired. Start making note of your feelings whenever you find yourself thinking about grabbing a snack. You may find that most of the time, you just need to get moving, talk to a friend on the phone, or go to bed.

10. If you feel hungry, drink some water.

It's often very difficult to tell the difference between thirst and hunger. Anytime you feel the urge for a snack, drink a glass of water. You may find the hunger pangs disappear more often than not.

EXERCISE ON THE 5:2 FAST DIET

Exercise is essential for both overall health and healthy weight loss. You can lose eight pounds without exercise, but you still might not like the results. We've all seen thin men and women who looked soft, pale, and flabby. The purpose of losing weight should be to look fit and healthy and to feel strong and energetic. That requires not only good nutrition but regular exercise as well.

A complete exercise program needs to include both cardio activity and some form of strength training. Cardio helps you to burn calories, improves cardiovascular health, and can also help with high blood pressure and type 2 diabetes. Strength training builds lean muscle (which helps you burn more calories throughout the day), improves bone health, and has been shown to improve longevity.

You should aim to get at least thirty minutes of cardio activity three times per week and at least twenty minutes of strength training three times per week. These are minimums and you can certainly do more, but if your schedule is tight you can get a great workout in less than thirty minutes.

Interval Training for Fast Results in Less Time

One way to get fast results in a very short time is through interval training. Interval training is simply alternating periods of physical work. You can do this to combine strength training with cardio or use it for cardio alone. For instance:

- Do three sets of bench presses, followed by two minutes of jumping rope, followed by three sets of biceps curls, and so on.
- Walk on a flat terrain for five minutes and then walk up two flights of stairs. Then walk on flat terrain for another five minutes, and so on.
- Alternate five laps using the breaststroke with five laps using the backstroke stroke and so on.

High-Intensity Interval Training

High-intensity interval training (HIIT) is a variation of interval training that is much more effective, but also much more intense. It's a cardio workout that can get you incredible results in just a few minutes per day, but it's not for everyone.

With high-intensity interval training, you alternate very short bursts of very hard work with longer periods of more moderate work.

The high-intensity intervals generally last from ten to thirty seconds and the moderate periods from two to four minutes. Almost any cardio activity can be adapted to high-intensity interval training. You can run at a moderate pace for two minutes, sprint for thirty seconds, and then go back to running. Repeat this pattern for a total of about twenty minutes, beginning and ending with a moderate period. You can also adapt HIIT to cycling, stair climbing, and several other cardio activities in which it's easy to change your pace.

HIIT has been shown to have a huge impact on metabolism. You can expect to burn more calories (even when you're resting) for about forty-eight hours after a HIIT workout. HIIT workouts also typically burn as many calories in twenty minutes as sixty minutes of the same activity in the steady-state version.

Whether you choose to do interval training or not, be sure to get at least three strength training workouts and three cardio workouts per week. You can do these on the same day or on alternating days, but as you'll soon read, strenuous exercise is not recommended on fasting days. Schedule your workouts so that you can get by with a moderate walk or some stretching on your fasting days. Cardio doesn't have to be tough to be good for you.

Some good cardio choices are walking, swimming, cycling, dancing, and rowing. Strength training can be done at home or the gym, with weight machines or dumbbells. You can also get a complete and effective workout using body-weight resistance moves such as push-ups, pull-ups, lunges, and the like.

You may want to get through your first week or two of the 5:2 Fast Diet before you commit to a regular workout program. It will be helpful for you to know more about how your body adjusts to the diet, how you feel on fasting days, and what times of day may be best for you to work out. Most people report improved energy levels and strength when following an intermittent fasting diet, but everyone adjusts to the diet in their own time. Until then, a thirty-minute walk or some stretching exercises will still do your body good.

Exercise on Fasting Days

Although you've probably read or heard assertions that you can continue doing intense workouts even on fasting days, we don't recommend it—at least not in the first few weeks of the 5:2 Fast Diet.

Our bodies are extremely adaptable mechanisms, but each body adapts in its own timeframe. While one person's metabolism may adjust itself to sourcing stored energy (in the form of stored fat) more readily, others may take longer. This is due to differences in eating and exercise habits prior to starting the diet, as well as hormone fluctuations.

On fasting days, you're eating enough to function and even function well, but you may not have the stored energy from non-fasting days or from stored fat to support a strenuous workout. The most benign result would be that you simply lack the energy or strength to perform the workout to a standard that makes it worthwhile. Even if you do get through your workout, you might find yourself far hungrier than you should be afterward.

More serious effects of working out too hard on fasting days could range from dizziness or feeling faint to muscle cramping or even injury.

On fasting days, we recommend that you do get some physical exercise, but only at an easy or moderate level. This might mean swimming laps at a moderate pace, taking a thirty-minute walk, or doing yoga or stretching exercises.

All physical activity is good for your body and will help you lose weight. Keep your strenuous workouts for non-fasting days and give your body a bit of a break when you're fasting.

OTHER HEALTH BENEFITS OF THE 5:2 FAST DIET

Although many people undertake intermittent fasting and the 5:2 Fast Diet in order to lose weight or to help maintain weight, there are many other health benefits. Since the goal of weight loss should be not only to look better but to improve overall health, these benefits should be considered just as important as losing fat or fitting into smaller clothes.

Research about the effects of intermittent fasting is ongoing, but numerous studies indicate that intermittent fasting can have a significant impact on longevity, cognitive function, heart disease, and blood sugar-related issues such as insulin sensitivity and metabolic syndrome.

Insulin- and Blood Sugar-Related Benefits of Intermittent Fasting

In a 2005 study conducted in Denmark, eight healthy men were put on a program of alternate-day fasting for fifteen days. At the end of the fifteen days, the men showed a marked improvement in their insulin sensitivity. The researchers explained that this improvement correlated with the theory of the "thrifty gene," which is that in the Paleolithic era, man frequently had to go days without eating, so our genes adapted to this feast or famine lifestyle. Specifically, certain hormones, such as *cortisol*, stimulate fat storage to get us by in times of little food.

The researchers commented that the abundance of food today has meant that we don't undergo fasting periods and this has contributed to the rise of metabolic syndrome or the combination of insulin resistance and obesity (Halberg N et al, 2005). They reported: "This experiment is the first in humans to show that intermittent fasting increases insulin-mediated glucose uptake rates, and the findings are compatible with the thrifty gene concept."

This study is one of several that suggest the process of fasting is necessary in order to help regulate insulin sensitivity and the ability of the body to use glucose as fuel instead of storing it as fat.

A 2011 study directed by Dr. Benjamin Horne, PhD, MPH, and the director of cardiovascular and genetic epidemiology at the Intermountain Medical Center Heart Institute, found that intermittent fasting had a positive impact on both cholesterol and human growth hormone (HGH) levels.

The study found that intermittent fasting raised the subjects' total cholesterol. LDL (low-density lipoprotein) or "bad" cholesterol was raised by 14 percent and HDL (high-density lipoprotein) or "good" cholesterol was raised by 6 percent. At first, this may seem like a bad thing, but as Dr. Horne explained, higher total cholesterol actually helps the body utilize fat as energy, which lowers overall body fat. The study further clarified: "Fasting causes hunger or stress. In response, the body releases more cholesterol, allowing it to utilize fat as a source of fuel, instead of glucose. This decreases the number of fat cells in the body, which is important because the fewer fat cells a body has, the less likely it will experience insulin resistance, or diabetes" (Horne BD et al, 2011).

These studies are just the tip of the iceberg in proving that intermittent fasting plans, such as the 5:2 Fast Diet, can have long-term benefits for insulin and blood sugar.

Intermittent Fasting and Heart Disease

Reducing fat and regulating blood sugar and insulin levels are both significant steps to better heart health. But there have been studies that show intermittent fasting can improve heart health and decrease risk of coronary artery disease in other ways as well. One such study was conducted by Dr. Benjamin Horne. In 2012, a study published in the *American Journal of Cardiology* found that periodic fasting may decrease the risk of both type 2 diabetes and coronary artery disease (Horne BD et al, 2012). These results are promising for those looking to reduce risk of heart disease through intermittent fasting.

Intermittent Fasting and Brain Health

Mark Mattson of the National Institute on Aging has done a great deal of research on intermittent fasting. His findings suggest that intermittent fasting boosts the production of *brain-derived neurotrophic factor* (BDNF), which is a protein that stimulates brain stem cells to become new neurons. It also protects brain cells from neurological degenerative disorders such as Alzheimer's and Parkinson's disease. According to Mattson's research, intermittent fasting can boost the production of BDNF by anywhere from 50 to 400 percent. In a 2012 *Washington Post* interview, he discussed the findings on fasting and Alzheimer's: "In mice engineered to develop Alzheimer's-like symptoms, alternate-day fasting begun in middle age delayed the onset of memory problems by about six months. This is a large effect, perhaps equivalent to 20 years in humans" (Young, 2012).

Everyone wants to be attractive, to feel fit, and to be more confident in their own skin. These are all things that can be accomplished with the help of the 5:2 Fast Diet. However, the possible long-term and very significant health benefits could be considered the primary appeal of the diet.

FASTING-DAY RECIPES

> **Note on Fasting-Day Recipes:** All of the fasting-day recipes were created to make two servings. If you don't have a friend or family member following the 5:2 Fast Diet with you, simply halve the recipe or save the second portion for another meal.

#1: Greek Breakfast Wraps (250 calories per serving)

This recipe is just as satisfying as that fast-food breakfast sandwich, but this wrap has far less fat and fewer calories. It's a great breakfast to make ahead of time and reheat in the morning or when you get to work.

- 1 teaspoon olive oil
- ½ cup fresh baby spinach leaves
- 1 tablespoon fresh basil
- 4 egg whites, beaten
- ½ teaspoon salt
- ¼ teaspoon freshly ground black pepper
- ¼ cup crumbed low-fat feta cheese
- 2 (8-inch) whole wheat tortillas

In a small skillet, heat the olive oil over medium heat. Add the spinach and basil to the pan and sauté for about 2 minutes, or just until the spinach is wilted.

Add the egg whites to the pan, season with the salt and pepper, and sauté, stirring often, for about 2 minutes more, or until the egg whites are firm.

Remove from the heat and sprinkle with the feta cheese.

Heat the tortillas in the microwave for 20 to 30 seconds, or just until softened and warm.

Divide the eggs between the tortillas and wrap up burrito-style.

Yields 2 servings.

#2: Parmesan Egg Toast with Tomatoes (150 calories per serving)

This breakfast is quick to make and delicious to eat. You can substitute grape tomatoes if you have them on hand. They provide a healthy dose of vitamin C to your meal.

- 1 teaspoon olive oil
- ½ teaspoon chopped garlic (about 1 clove)
- 6 cherry tomatoes, quartered
- ½ teaspoon salt
- ¼ teaspoon freshly ground black pepper
- 2 large eggs
- 2 slices reduced-calorie whole wheat toast
- 1 tablespoon shredded Parmesan cheese

In a small skillet, heat the olive oil over medium heat. Add the garlic and tomatoes to the pan and sauté for 2 minutes, stirring often. Season with the salt and pepper, then transfer to a plate to keep warm.

In the same skillet, fry the eggs for 2 minutes. Turn over and cook to the desired doneness (30 seconds for over easy, 1 minute for over medium, 2 minutes for over well).

Place 1 egg on each slice of toast, top with half the tomatoes, and sprinkle with half the Parmesan cheese.

Yields 2 servings.

#3: Curried Chicken Breast Wraps (250 calories per serving)

These quick and filling wraps deliver a lot of flavor for very few calories. Make the filling ahead of time to have on hand for work lunches and busy days.

- 6 ounces cooked chicken breast, cubed
- 2 tablespoons plain low-fat yogurt
- 1 teaspoon Dijon mustard
- ½ teaspoon mild curry powder
- 1 small Gala or Granny Smith apple, cored and chopped
- 1 cup spring lettuce mix or baby lettuce
- 2 (8-inch) whole wheat tortillas

In a small bowl, combine the chicken, yogurt, Dijon mustard, and curry powder; stir well to combine. Add the apple and stir until blended.

Divide the lettuce between the tortillas and top each with half of the chicken mixture. Roll up burrito-style and serve.

Yields 2 servings.

#4: Baked Salmon Fillets with Tomato and Mushrooms (200 calories per serving)

Salmon is a great source of healthy fats, especially omega-3 fatty acids. When baked with a mixture of tangy tomatoes and mild mushrooms, it's as delicious as it is healthy.

- 2 (4-ounce) skin-on salmon fillets
- 2 teaspoons olive oil, divided
- ½ teaspoon salt
- ¼ teaspoon freshly ground black pepper
- ½ teaspoon chopped fresh dill
- ½ cup diced fresh tomato
- ½ cup sliced fresh mushrooms

Preheat the oven to 375 degrees F and line a baking sheet with aluminum foil.

Using your fingers or a pastry brush, coat both sides of the fillets with ½ teaspoon of the olive oil each. Place the salmon skin-side down on the pan. Sprinkle evenly with the salt and pepper.

In a small bowl, combine the remaining 1 teaspoon olive oil, the dill, tomato, and mushrooms; stir well to combine. Spoon the mixture over the fillets.

Fold the sides and ends of the foil up to seal the fish, place the pan on the middle oven rack, and bake for about 20 minutes, or until the salmon flakes easily.

Yields 2 servings.

#5: Protein Power Sweet Potatoes (200 calories per serving)

This recipe is extremely simple and quick, but it packs almost ten grams of protein per serving, which makes it a perfect fasting-day meal for keeping you full and helping you stay energized and focused.

- 2 medium sweet potatoes
- ½ teaspoon salt
- ¼ teaspoon freshly ground black pepper
- 6 ounces plain Greek yogurt
- ⅓ cup dried cranberries

Preheat the oven to 400 degrees F and pierce the sweet potatoes several times with a fork. Place them on a baking sheet dish and bake for 40 to 45 minutes, or until easily pierced with a fork.

Cut the potatoes in half and spoon the flesh into a medium mixing bowl, keeping the skins intact. Add the salt, pepper, yogurt, and cranberries to the bowl and mix well with a fork.

Spoon the mixture back into the potato skins and serve warm.

Yields 2 servings.

#6: Avocado and Fennel Salad with Balsamic Vinaigrette (150 calories per serving)

This salad is a wonderful blend of tangy citrus, silky avocado, and anise-flavored fennel. Tossed with a quick and easy balsamic vinaigrette, it's a perfect lunch or light supper for warm days.

- 1 tablespoon light olive oil
- 1 tablespoon balsamic vinegar
- ¼ teaspoon salt
- ¼ teaspoon freshly ground black pepper
- ½ cup fennel, sliced
- ½ avocado, diced
- ½ cup mandarin oranges, drained
- 1 cup chopped romaine lettuce

In a medium mixing bowl, combine the olive oil, balsamic vinegar, salt, and pepper, and whisk until well combined and slightly thickened. This is your balsamic vinaigrette.

Add the fennel, avocado, oranges, and lettuce; toss until the vegetables are well coated with dressing. Divide between two salad plates and serve cold.

Yields 2 servings.

#7: Penne Pasta with Vegetables (200 calories per serving)

Even on fasting days, you can enjoy a light pasta meal. This one is chock-full of vitamin C and iron from the spinach and tomatoes and delivers lots of flavor and satisfaction.

- 1 teaspoon salt, divided
- ¾ cup uncooked penne pasta
- 1 tablespoon olive oil
- 1 tablespoon chopped garlic
- 1 teaspoon chopped fresh oregano
- 1 cup sliced fresh mushrooms
- 10 cherry tomatoes, halved
- 1 cup fresh spinach leaves
- ½ teaspoon freshly ground black pepper
- 1 tablespoon shredded Parmesan cheese

In a large saucepan, bring 1 quart water to a boil. Add ½ teaspoon of the salt and the penne, and cook according to package directions, or until al dente (about 9 minutes). Drain but do not rinse the penne, reserving about ¼ cup pasta water.

Meanwhile, in a large skillet, heat the olive oil over medium-high heat. Add the garlic, oregano, and mushrooms, and sauté for 4 to 5 minutes, or until the mushrooms are golden.

Add the tomatoes and spinach, season with the remaining ½ teaspoon salt and the black pepper, and sauté for 3 to 4 minutes, or until the spinach is wilted.

Add the drained pasta to the skillet, along with 2 to 3 tablespoons of the pasta water. Cook, stirring constantly, for 2 to 3 minutes, or until the pasta is glistening and the water has cooked off.

Divide the pasta between two shallow bowls and sprinkle with the Parmesan cheese. Serve hot or at room temperature.

Yields 2 servings.

#8: Hearty Shrimp and Kale Soup (250 calories per serving)

This tasty soup packs plenty of antioxidants from the carrots and kale, plus a healthy amount of protein from the shrimp and beans. It's delicious, simple, and satisfying.

- 1 teaspoon olive oil
- 2 cloves garlic
- ¼ cup chopped onion
- 2 cups chopped fresh kale
- 1 cup thinly sliced fresh carrots
- ½ teaspoon salt
- ¼ teaspoon freshly ground black pepper
- 1½ cups vegetable stock
- 8 medium (36–40 count) raw shrimp, peeled and halved
- 1 cup canned great northern beans, drained
- ¼ cup chopped fresh parsley

In a medium saucepan, heat the olive oil over medium heat. Add the garlic, onion, kale, and carrots, and sauté for 5 minutes, stirring often.

Season the vegetables with the salt and pepper, then add the vegetable stock. Simmer, uncovered, for 30 minutes, or until the carrots are fork-tender.

Increase the heat to high and bring the soup to a boil. Add the shrimp and cook for 2 minutes, or until the shrimp are pink and somewhat firm. Reduce the heat to low.

Use a fork to mash about one-quarter of the beans. Stir all the beans into the soup and add the parsley. Simmer for 2 minutes, or until heated through.

Ladle into soup bowls and serve hot.

Yields 2 servings.

#9: Pork Loin Chops with Mango Salsa (250 calories per serving)

This recipe is bursting with flavor and is satisfying enough to make you forget that you're fasting. The salsa is even better made a day ahead, so allow it to marinate in the fridge overnight with the pork chops.

- 2 pork loin chops, ¾ inch thick
- ½ cup lime juice
- Juice of 1 large orange
- 1 large just ripe mango, peeled and diced
- ½ cup diced red onion
- ½ cup diced green bell pepper
- ½ cup diced red bell pepper
- 1 small jalapeño pepper, seeded and diced
- 1 tablespoon chopped fresh cilantro
- 1 tablespoon chopped fresh parsley
- ½ teaspoon salt
- ¼ teaspoon freshly ground black pepper

Place the pork chops in a freezer bag and add the lime and orange juices. Seal, shake to mix well, and place in the refrigerator overnight.

In a small bowl, combine the mango, red onion, bell peppers, jalapeño, cilantro, and parsley. Stir to combine very well. Cover and refrigerate overnight.

Preheat the broiler and line a baking pan with aluminum foil.

Season each pork chop on both sides with the salt and pepper. Place on the pan and broil for 4 to 5 minutes on one side, then turn over and broil for 4 to 5 minutes more.

Place each pork chop on a plate, spoon the salsa over the top, and serve.

Yields 2 servings.

#10: Lemon-Sesame Chicken and Asparagus (200 calories per serving)

Chicken and asparagus go together beautifully, and this recipe combines them with a hint of lemon and the added crunch of sesame seeds.

- 8 ounces skinless chicken breast tenders (or quartered chicken breast)
- ½ cup plus 1 tablespoon lemon juice, divided
- 1 teaspoon salt, divided
- ¼ teaspoon freshly ground black pepper
- 1 teaspoon chopped fresh rosemary
- 6 medium spears fresh asparagus, cut into 2-inch pieces
- ½ teaspoon olive oil
- 2 tablespoons sesame seeds

Pound out the chicken tenders with a mallet or the heel of your hand until they are a uniform ½ inch thickness. Place in a freezer bag with the ½ cup lemon juice and marinate for 2 hours or overnight.

Preheat the broiler and line a baking pan with aluminum foil.

Season the chicken on both sides with ½ teaspoon of the salt and the pepper, and place on the pan. Sprinkle with the rosemary.

In a small bowl, toss the asparagus with the olive oil, remaining 1 tablespoon lemon juice, and remaining ½ teaspoon salt. Arrange the asparagus around the chicken on the pan.

Broil the chicken for 4 to 5 minutes, then turn it over and stir the asparagus, and broil for 4 to 5 minutes more.

Divide the chicken and asparagus between two plates and sprinkle with the sesame seeds.

Yields 2 servings.

#11: Spinach and Swiss Cheese Omelet (150 calories per serving)

Omelets don't need to be reserved for breakfast or brunch. An omelet can be a great dinner solution on busy nights and also makes a satisfying lunch entrée on weekends.

- 1 teaspoon olive oil
- 1 cup fresh baby spinach leaves
- ½ teaspoon salt
- ¼ teaspoon freshly ground black pepper
- 6 large egg whites, beaten
- 2 (1-ounce) slices reduced-fat Swiss cheese

In a small skillet, heat the olive oil over medium-high heat. Add the spinach, salt, and pepper, and sauté for 3 minutes, stirring often.

Use a spatula to spread the spinach fairly evenly over the bottom of the pan, and pour the egg whites over the top, tilting the pan to coat the spinach completely.

Cook for 3 to 4 minutes, occasionally pulling the edges of the eggs toward the center as you tilt the skillet to allow uncooked egg to spread to the edges of the pan.

When the center of the eggs are mostly (but not completely) dry, use a spatula to flip the eggs. Place the Swiss cheese slices on one half of the omelet, and then flip the other half over the top to form a half moon. Cook for 1 minute, or until the cheese is melted and warm.

To serve, cut the omelet in half and serve hot.

Yields 2 servings.

#12: Grilled Chicken Salad with Poppy Seed Dressing (200 calories per serving)

Salads are easy to put together, and when made with lots of fresh, high-fiber vegetables, they provide lots of food for very few calories. This salad not only tastes great but also fills you up nicely, too.

- 2 tablespoons light olive oil
- 1 tablespoon apple cider vinegar
- 1 teaspoon Dijon mustard
- 1 tablespoon poppy seeds
- ½ cup chopped cooked chicken breast
- 1 cup chopped romaine lettuce
- 1 medium unpeeled cucumber, sliced
- 1 medium red bell pepper, chopped
- 1 small red onion, chopped

In a medium mixing bowl, whisk together the olive oil, cider vinegar, Dijon mustard, and poppy seeds for about 1 minute, or until well blended and smooth.

Add the chicken, lettuce, cucumber, bell pepper, and onion, and toss well until evenly coated.

Divide between two salad plates and serve immediately.

Yields 2 servings.

#13: Quick Miso Soup with Bok Choy and Shrimp (150 calories per serving)

If you enjoy Asian flavors, you'll love this simple, quick soup. It comes together in just a few minutes, making it a great recipe for your busiest nights. It reheats well, so it's also a good choice for a workday lunch.

- 2 cups water
- 8 large (34–40 count) raw shrimp, peeled and halved
- 1 cup chopped bok choy
- ¼ cup white miso paste
- 1 cup cubed firm tofu
- 2 green onions, chopped

In a medium saucepan, bring the water to a boil over high heat. Add the shrimp and boil for 1 minute.

Reduce the heat to low and stir in the bok choy. Simmer for 2 minutes, then stir in the miso and tofu. Simmer for 1 minute more.

To serve, divide between two soup bowls and sprinkle with the green onions.

Yields 2 servings.

#14: Broiled Halibut with Garlic Spinach (200 calories per serving)

Halibut is a deliciously moist fish that is loaded with heart-healthy omega-3 fatty acids. If you substitute frozen halibut, be sure to thaw it completely and pat it very dry before cooking.

- 2 (4-ounce) halibut fillets, 1 inch thick
- ½ lemon (about 1 teaspoon juice)
- 1 teaspoon salt, divided
- ¼ teaspoon freshly ground black pepper
- ½ teaspoon cayenne pepper
- 1 teaspoon olive oil
- 2 cloves garlic
- ½ cup chopped red onion
- 2 cups fresh baby spinach leaves

Preheat the broiler and place an oven rack 4 to 5 inches below the heat source. Line a baking sheet with aluminum foil.

Squeeze the lemon half over the fish fillets, then season each side with ½ teaspoon of the salt, pepper, and cayenne. Place the fish on the pan and broil for 7 to 8 minutes. Turn over the fish and broil for 6 to 7 minutes more, or until flaky.

Meanwhile, heat the olive oil in a small skillet over medium heat. Add the garlic and onion, and sauté for 2 minutes. Add the spinach and remaining ½ teaspoon salt, and sauté for 2 minutes more. Remove from the heat and cover to keep warm.

To serve, divide the spinach between two plates and top each portion with a fish fillet. Serve hot.

Yields 2 servings.

#15: Quinoa with Curried Black Beans and Sweet Potatoes (250 calories per serving)

The beans, quinoa, and sweet potatoes combine to deliver a healthy and filling portion of meatless protein that is very satisfying. You can prepare the quinoa in the microwave if you prefer; just follow package directions to yield one cup.

- ½ cup quinoa
- 1 cup water
- ½ cup peeled and diced sweet potato (about 1 small)
- ½ teaspoon olive oil
- ½ teaspoon dried rosemary
- 1 cup canned black beans, drained
- 1 teaspoon mild curry powder
- 2 tablespoons chopped fresh parsley

Rinse the quinoa under cold running water in a fine mesh sieve. Drain very well over paper towels and then pat dry.

In a small saucepan, toast the quinoa for 2 minutes over medium heat, shaking frequently. Add the water, increase the heat to high, and bring the water to a boil. Cover, reduce the heat to low, and cook for 15 minutes, or until the quinoa is plump and the germ forms little spirals on each grain. Remove from the heat and cover to keep warm.

In a small bowl, toss the sweet potato with the olive oil and rosemary. Transfer to a medium skillet over medium-high heat. Sauté, stirring frequently, for 6 to 7 minutes, or until well caramelized. Stir in the black beans and curry powder, reduce the heat to medium, and cook, stirring frequently, until the beans are heated through.

To serve, place ½ cup cooked quinoa on each plate and top with half of the bean mixture. Garnish with the parsley.

Yields 2 servings.

#16: Toasted Pepper Jack Sandwiches (150 calories per serving)

Toasting, rather than grilling, your cheese sandwich adds tons of satisfying crunch while omitting extra fat. These toasted cheese sandwiches pack a lot of spicy flavor into every bite.

- 2 slices reduced-calorie pepper jack cheese
- 4 slices reduced-calorie whole wheat bread
- ½ cup fresh arugula leaves
- 4 thin slices fresh tomato

Preheat the oven to 350 degrees F.

Place 1 slice of cheese on each of 2 slices of bread; top each with 2 slices of tomato and half of the arugula. Top with the remaining bread slices and put the sandwiches on a baking sheet in the center of the oven.

Toast for 4 minutes, then turn over and toast for 2 to 3 minutes more, or until the bread is golden and the cheese is melted. Cut each sandwich in half to serve.

Yields 2 servings.

ONE-MONTH FASTING-DAY MEAL PLAN

Each fasting day includes two of the recipes from Chapter 6, plus delicious snacks from the list that follows. Women will eat 500 calories per day, while men will eat 600 calories per day.

You are not restricted to eating breakfast foods for breakfast or dinner foods for dinner. You're free to switch your meals around. For instance, on Week One, Day #1, you'll have Parmesan Egg Toast with Tomatoes, a Curried Chicken Breast Wrap, and snacks totaling either 100 calories (for women) or 200 calories (for men). If you'd like to eat a snack for breakfast and have the meals for lunch and dinner, that's fine. If you'd like to have the Parmesan Egg Toast for breakfast, the chicken wrap for dinner, and your snacks during the day in between, that's also fine. For this reason, the meal plans are not broken up into specific times of day, but instead into meals and snacks. This makes it much easier to plan your fasting-day meals around your schedule and helps keep you from falling off track.

Each fasting day, you'll have two meals and two snacks. ***Men simply need to double the portions of the snacks to get the required number of daily calories.*** Feel free to choose items in the 50-Calorie Supplemental Food and Snack List below that appeal to you.

On all fasting days, allowed beverages are limited to water, unsweetened hot or iced tea, and black coffee.

Week 1 Plan

Fasting Day 1

First Meal (150 calories): Parmesan Egg Toast with Tomatoes (#2)

Second Meal (250 calories): Curried Chicken Breast Wrap (#3)

Snacks (50 calories each): ½ medium apple, baked and sprinkled with cinnamon; 1 slice crispbread with 1 ounce cottage cheese

Fasting Day 2

First Meal (200 calories): Protein Power Sweet Potatoes (#5)

Second Meal (200 calories): Lemon-Sesame Chicken and Asparagus (#10)

Snacks (50 calories each): ½ medium frozen banana; 1 mini-box raisins

Week 2 Plan

Fasting Day 1

First Meal (200 calories): Grilled Chicken Salad with Poppy Seed Dressing (#12)

Second Meal (200 calories): Baked Salmon Fillets with Tomato and Mushrooms (#4)

Snacks (50 calories each): 4 ounces unsweetened applesauce sprinkled with cinnamon; 1½ cups air-popped popcorn

Fasting Day 2

First Meal (250 calories): Hearty Shrimp and Kale Soup (#8)

Second Meal (150 calories): Spinach and Swiss Cheese Omelet (#11)

Snacks (50 calories each): ½ cup strawberries with 2 tablespoons fat-free vanilla yogurt; ½ cup shelled edamame with sea salt

Week 3 Plan

Fasting Day 1

First Meal (250 calories): Quinoa with Curried Black Beans and Sweet Potatoes (#15)

Second Meal (150 calories): Quick Miso Soup with Bok Choy and Shrimp (#13)

Snacks (50 calories each): 1 medium peach; 2 tablespoons hummus with 2 slices red bell pepper

Fasting Day 2

First Meal (200 calories): Broiled Halibut with Garlic Spinach (#14)

Second Meal (200 calories): Penne Pasta with Vegetables (#7)

Snacks (50 calories each): 1 small celery stalk with ½ tablespoon almond butter; 2 slices avocado with lime juice

Week 4 Plan

Fasting Day 1

First Meal (250 calories): Greek Breakfast Wrap (#1)

Second Meal (150 calories): Avocado and Fennel Salad with Balsamic Vinaigrette (#6)

Snacks (50 calories each): 10 frozen grapes; 1 light Babybel cheese

Fasting Day 2

First Meal (250 calories): Pork Loin Chop with Mango Salsa (#9),

Second Meal (150 calories): Toasted Pepper Jack Sandwiches (#16)

Snacks (50 calories each): 12 cherries; ½ small apple with 1 teaspoon almond butter

The 50-Calorie Supplemental Food and Snack List

Your fasting-day meals will be rounded out with healthy foods from this list. Each of these items is 50 calories or just a bit less. Men should simply double the portions to achieve their higher daily intake needs (600 calories total).

You can also use this list to round out non-fasting-day meal plans you create with the healthy recipes in Chapters 8, 9, and 10. This simple way of calorie counting and portion control makes it much easier to stick with your plan long-term.

- Apple: ½ medium, baked and sprinkled with cinnamon
- Apple: ½ small, with 1 teaspoon almond butter
- Apple (Granny Smith): 1 small
- Applesauce (unsweetened): 4 ounces, sprinkled with cinnamon
- Avocado: 2 slices, with lime juice
- Babybel cheese (light): 1 round
- Baby carrots: ½ cup, with 1 tablespoon fat-free ranch
- Banana: ½ medium, frozen
- Blueberries ½ cup, with 2 teaspoons fat-free plain yogurt
- Brown rice cake: 1 cake, with ½ teaspoon almond butter
- Cantaloupe (chopped): ½ cup, with 2 tablespoons fat-free cottage cheese
- Celery stalk: 1 small, with ½ tablespoon almond butter
- Cherries: 12 whole
- Cherry tomatoes: 16 whole
- Crispbread: 1 slice, with 1 ounce cottage cheese

- Dill pickles: 6 medium

- Edamame (shelled): ½ cup, with sea salt

- Grapes (frozen): 10 whole

- Greek yogurt (fat-free): ½ cup, with ½ cup blueberries

- Green olives (pitted): 10 whole

- Hummus: 2 tablespoons, with 2 slices red bell pepper

- Miso soup (instant): 1 cup, with ¼ cup frozen spinach

- Peach: 1 medium

- Popcorn (air popped): 1½ cups

- Raisins: 1 mini-box

- Red grapefruit: ½ large

- Strawberries: ½ cup, with 2 tablespoons fat-free vanilla yogurt

- Strawberries: 12 whole

- Tangerine: 1 whole

- Tomato: 1 large, with 1 tablespoon Parmesan cheese

- Turkey breast: 2 (1-ounce) slices, wrapped in leaf lettuce

- Vegetable juice blend: 6 ounces

HEALTHY RECIPES FOR NON-FASTING DAYS: BREAKFAST

Note on Non-Fasting Day Recipes: The recipes for non-fasting days are low in calories but suitable for guests or the entire family, so we've created most of them to make four servings. If you like, you can either halve the ingredients or freeze extra servings for easy reheating on another day.

Nutty Peach Parfaits

These parfaits may look pretty, but they're even healthier than they look. The walnuts add omega-3 fats and fiber as well as crunch, and the Greek yogurt has as much as fourteen grams of protein per cup.

- 4 medium peaches, sliced
- 4 (6-ounce) containers vanilla Greek yogurt
- ½ cup unsalted walnuts, chopped

Divide the ingredients between four parfait or dessert dishes. Start with a layer of peaches; then add a spoonful of yogurt and then a sprinkling of walnuts.

Yields 4 servings.

Salmon and Tomato Egg Sandwiches

This breakfast sandwich is far healthier and more substantial than anything you can pick up at the drive-through; it's also a lot tastier, but only takes a few minutes to prepare.

- 4 light multigrain English muffins
- 1 teaspoon olive oil
- 6 ounces canned pink salmon
- 1 cup diced tomatoes
- 8 large eggs, beaten
- ½ teaspoon salt
- ¼ teaspoon freshly ground black pepper
- 1 cup fresh arugula

Toast the English muffins while you prepare the eggs.

In a medium skillet, heat the olive oil over medium-high heat. Add the salmon and tomatoes to the pan, and sauté, stirring frequently, for 4 minutes.

Pour the eggs over the top, season with the salt and pepper, and scramble, stirring frequently, for about 2 minutes, or until the eggs are set.

Place the English muffin halves on 4 plates and top each bottom half with one-quarter of the egg mixture. Top with arugula and the other muffin half.

Yields 4 servings.

Cocoa-Banana Breakfast Smoothie

This smoothie takes just seconds to make, but it's loaded with nutrition. The Greek yogurt provides a healthy dose of protein and the bananas are a great source of potassium.

- 24 ounces vanilla Greek yogurt
- 2 medium bananas, cut into chunks
- 1 teaspoon honey
- 2 tablespoons unsweetened cocoa powder
- ½ cup low-fat milk
- ½ cup ice cubes

Place the yogurt and bananas into a blender and blend on high until the bananas are smooth.

Add the honey, cocoa, and milk and blend again until well incorporated.

Add the ice and blend again, pulsing as needed, until the mixture is smooth and thick.

Yields 4 servings.

Cranberry-Walnut Whole Wheat Pancakes

These pancakes are a delicious way to start your day. The cranberries are tart yet sweet, and the walnuts add crunch and texture to this comfort classic.

- ½ cup fresh cranberries
- ¾ cup whole wheat flour
- 2 tablespoons sugar
- 1 tablespoon baking powder
- ¼ teaspoon salt
- ½ teaspoon ground nutmeg
- ½ teaspoon pure vanilla extract
- 1¼ cup low-fat milk
- 1 large egg, beaten
- ½ cup chopped walnuts
- 1 tablespoon coconut oil, divided

In a small bowl, combine the cranberries with a handful of the whole wheat flour, tossing them well to coat.

In a large mixing bowl, combine the remaining flour, sugar, baking powder, salt, and nutmeg, stirring to blend well.

Add the vanilla, milk, and egg and stir to blend, but don't overmix. The batter should remain somewhat lumpy. Gently fold in the walnuts and cranberries (with flour) and set the batter aside for 10 minutes.

In a large heavy skillet, heat about ½ teaspoon of the coconut oil over medium heat. Ladle enough batter into the pan to make a 6-inch pancake. Cook for about 2 minutes, or until the edges are bubbly, then flip the pancake and cook for 1 minute more. Transfer to a plate and cover to keep warm while you make the rest of the pancakes. Add additional coconut oil to the pan as needed.

To serve, place 2 pancakes on each plate and top with warm maple syrup, honey, or molasses.

Yields 4 servings.

Scrambled Egg Soft Tacos

Finding alternatives to fast food for your morning meal can be a challenge, but this recipe is an excellent one to try. It's loaded with southwestern flavor, but low in both fat and calories.

- 8 (6-inch) whole wheat tortillas
- 1 teaspoon olive oil
- 2 green onions, chopped
- ½ teaspoon cayenne pepper
- 12 large eggs, beaten
- 1 cup mild chunky salsa
- 1 cup low-fat shredded cheddar cheese

Place the tortillas on a plate, top with a damp paper towel, and microwave for 30 to 45 seconds, or just until warm and pliable. Cover with a second plate or pot lid to keep warm.

In a large heavy skillet, heat the olive oil over medium heat. Add the green onions and sauté for 1 minute. Stir the cayenne into the eggs, then pour them into the skillet. Scramble, stirring constantly, until the eggs are cooked, about 5 minutes.

Divide the egg mixture evenly between the tortillas, top the tortillas with 2 tablespoons each salsa and cheddar cheese, and fold the tacos in half.

Yields 4 servings (2 tacos each).

Herb and Swiss Frittata

This frittata looks like something you'd see in a restaurant, but it takes just a few minutes to prepare. You'll love the layered flavors, courtesy of mild Swiss cheese and fresh herbs.

- 2 teaspoons olive oil
- 8 large eggs, beaten
- ½ teaspoon salt
- ½ teaspoon freshly ground black pepper
- 2 teaspoons chopped fresh parsley
- 2 teaspoons chopped fresh marjoram
- 1 teaspoon chopped fresh basil
- ½ cup shredded low-fat Swiss cheese

Preheat the oven to 375 degrees F.

Heat the olive oil in a large ovenproof skillet over high heat. Pour in the eggs, distributing them evenly around the skillet. Season with the salt and pepper.

Remove the skillet from the heat and sprinkle the parsley, marjoram, and basil evenly over the top of the eggs. Top with the Swiss cheese.

Place the skillet in the middle of the oven and bake for 18 to 22 minutes, or until a toothpick inserted into the center comes out clean.

To serve, cut into four wedges and serve hot.

Yields 4 servings.

Vanilla-Almond Protein Shake

This breakfast shake has plenty of protein and healthy fats to keep you going on even your toughest mornings. This is a great way to get your breakfast to go—just pour into a travel mug and drink on your way.

- 2 cups cold water
- 4 scoops unflavored whey protein isolate powder
- ¼ cup almond butter
- 2 tablespoons honey
- ½ teaspoon almond extract
- ½ teaspoon ground nutmeg
- 10 ice cubes

In a blender, combine the cold water, protein powder, almond butter, honey, almond extract, and nutmeg. Blend on high for about 30 seconds, or until smooth.

Add the ice cubes and blend again until thick and creamy. Drink immediately.

Yields 2 servings.

Scrambled Eggs with Mushrooms and Onions

This egg dish cooks up in a hurry but has a flavor that will beg you to slow down and savor it. This makes a great sandwich filling, too. If you must eat breakfast on the run, a whole wheat pita pocket is a good choice.

- 1 teaspoon olive oil
- 1 cup sliced fresh mushrooms
- ¼ cup thinly sliced yellow onion
- 1 tablespoon chopped fresh tarragon
- ½ cup chopped fresh parsley
- ½ teaspoon salt
- ½ teaspoon freshly ground black pepper
- 8 large eggs, beaten

In a large heavy skillet, heat the olive oil over medium heat. Add the mushrooms, onion, tarragon, parsley, salt, and pepper, and sauté for 4 minutes, stirring occasionally.

Pour in the eggs and scramble, stirring constantly, until they are cooked, about 2 minutes.

To serve, divide between 4 plates.

Yields 4 servings.

Grilled Fruit Salad

Fruit doesn't always have to be raw; in fact, grilling or broiling fresh fruit brings out its natural sugars and intensifies its flavor. Double the recipe and use the leftovers as a side dish for chicken or seafood.

- 8 slices fresh or canned (unsweetened) pineapple
- 4 fresh peaches or nectarines, pitted and sliced into 8 pieces each
- 8 (½-inch-thick) slices fresh honeydew melon
- 1 teaspoon honey, warmed for 30 seconds in microwave
- ½ teaspoon salt

Preheat the broiler and line a baking sheet with aluminum foil.

Spread the fruit in a single layer on the baking sheet and brush with the honey on both sides.

Sprinkle the salt over the top and place the pan 3 inches below the broiler.

Broil for 3 minutes, turn each piece of fruit, then broil for 2 minutes more, or just until the fruit is slightly browned at the edges.

Place 2 pineapple slices, 8 peach slices, and 2 melon slices onto each of 4 plates and serve warm.

Yields 4 servings.

Hearty Hot Cereal with Berries

Whole grains are not only great for your heart; they're also great for your waist. The high fiber content makes them filling and provides slow, steady energy for your day. The addition of berries and nuts in this recipe makes it especially hearty.

- 4 cups water
- ½ teaspoon salt
- 2 cups whole rolled oats
- ½ cup chopped walnuts
- 2 teaspoons flaxseed
- 2 tablespoons honey
- ½ cup fresh blueberries
- ½ cup fresh raspberries
- 1 cup low-fat milk

In a medium saucepan, bring the water to a boil over high heat and add the salt.

Stir in the oats, walnuts, and flaxseed, then reduce the heat to low and cover. Cook for 16 to 20 minutes, or until the oatmeal reaches the desired consistency.

Divide the oatmeal between 4 deep bowls and top each with 2 tablespoons of both blueberries and raspberries. Add ¼ cup milk to each bowl and serve.

Yields 4 servings.

Easy Granola Bars

This recipe is far better for you than any commercial granola bars, which are often laden with high-fructose corn syrup and less healthy grains. These bars bake up in a jiffy and will keep in an airtight container for up to one week—that is, if they last that long.

- 1 teaspoon coconut oil
- 1 cup pecan pieces
- 1 cup raw pumpkin seeds
- 1 cup chopped walnuts
- 1 cup dried cranberries
- 1 cup dried apricots, chopped
- 1 cup unsweetened coconut flakes

- ¼ cup coconut oil, melted
- ½ cup almond butter
- ½ cup raw honey
- ¼ teaspoon pure vanilla extract
- ½ teaspoon salt
- 1 teaspoon ground cinnamon

Preheat the oven to 325 degrees F. Grease a 9-by-13-inch baking pan with the 1 teaspoon of coconut oil and set aside.

In a large bowl, combine the pecans, pumpkin seeds, walnuts, cranberries, apricots, and coconut flakes, and toss to mix well.

In a small saucepan over low heat, combine the melted coconut oil, almond butter, honey, vanilla, salt, and cinnamon, and heat just until the honey is melted.

Transfer the nut mixture to the baking pan, pressing down to spread it evenly. Pour the honey mixture evenly over the top.

Bake for 35 to 40 minutes, or until golden. Let the mixture cool to room temperature before cutting into equal bars. Store in an airtight container for up to 1 week.

Yields 1 dozen bars.

Pecan-Banana Pops

A healthy breakfast doesn't necessarily have to be hot; in fact, this one is frozen. Make a bunch of these pops ahead of time and keep them in the freezer. They make an excellent after-school treat as well. Kids love them!

- 4 large just-ripe bananas
- 4 Popsicle sticks
- ½ cup almond butter
- 2 tablespoons raw honey
- ¾ cup chopped pecans

Peel and cut one end from each banana, and insert a Popsicle stick into the cut end.

In a small bowl, stir together the almond butter and honey, and heat in the microwave for 10 to 15 seconds, or just until the mixture is slightly thinned. Pour onto a sheet of wax paper or aluminum foil and spread with a spatula.

On another piece of wax paper or foil, spread the chopped pecans. Line a small baking sheet or large plate with a third piece of wax paper or foil.

Roll each banana first in the honey mixture until well coated, then in the nuts until completely covered, pressing down gently so the nuts adhere.

Place each finished banana onto the baking sheet. When all of the bananas have been coated, place the sheet in the freezer for at least 2 hours. For long-term storage, transfer the frozen bananas into a resealable plastic bag.

Yields 4 pops.

HEALTHY RECIPES FOR NON-FASTING DAYS: LUNCH

Note on Non-Fasting Day Recipes: The recipes for non-fasting days are low in calories but suitable for guests or the entire family, so we've created most of them to make four servings. If you like, you can either halve the ingredients or freeze extra servings for easy reheating on another day.

Shrimp and Cranberry Salad

Dried cranberries add a tart touch of flavor to this fresh shrimp salad. Using steamed shrimp from your seafood counter makes this a very fast lunch to prepare.

- 1 dozen large (26–30 count) cooked shrimp, peeled and deveined
- ¼ cup lime juice
- ¼ teaspoon ground cumin
- ¼ teaspoon paprika
- 2 cups chopped romaine lettuce
- ½ cup sliced red onion
- ½ yellow bell pepper, chopped
- ½ orange bell pepper, chopped
- ¼ cup dried cranberries
- ¼ cup of your favorite homemade or store-bought balsamic vinaigrette

In a small bowl, toss the shrimp with the lime juice, cumin, and paprika, and let them sit for 30 minutes in the refrigerator. Drain.

In a large bowl, combine the lettuce, onion, bell peppers, and cranberries until evenly combined.

Add the marinated shrimp and balsamic vinaigrette and toss again. Divide between 4 salad plates and serve.

Yields 4 servings.

Tuna and Bean Salad Pockets

This light but filling recipe is a great one for workday lunches. It packs well and the flavor gets better the longer it has a chance to sit, so prepare the salad the night before and pop it into a pita pocket and then into your lunch bag in the morning.

- 4 whole wheat pita pockets
- 1 (6-ounce) can tuna packed in water, drained
- ½ (15-ounce) can pinto beans, rinsed and drained
- ¼ cup diced white onion
- 2 tablespoons light mayonnaise
- 1 teaspoon spicy brown mustard
- ½ teaspoon celery seed
- ½ teaspoon freshly ground black pepper
- 1 cup chopped romaine lettuce

If the pitas are unsliced, slice them so that there is a pocket-like opening, being careful not to cut through the sides or bottoms.

In a small mixing bowl, combine the tuna, pinto beans, onion, mayonnaise, mustard, celery seed, and pepper; mix well.

Divide the lettuce between the pita pockets, then fill each one with one-quarter of the tuna salad.

Yields 4 servings.

Chicken Breast with Roasted Summer Veggies

This recipe reheats well, so prepare it on a weekend or in the evening and pack in individual containers to take for your lunch during the week. Experiment with other seasonal vegetables to vary the flavors.

- 4 (4- to 5-ounce) skinless chicken breasts
- 1 teaspoon plus 1 tablespoon olive oil, divided
- 1 teaspoon salt, divided
- ½ teaspoon freshly ground black pepper, divided
- ½ teaspoon ground turmeric
- 1 medium zucchini, thinly sliced
- 2 yellow squash, thinly sliced
- 1 medium white onion, sliced ½ inch thick
- 1 pint cherry tomatoes
- 1 teaspoon dried parsley
- 1 teaspoon dried oregano

Preheat the oven to 400 degrees F and line a baking pan with aluminum foil.

Rub both sides of the chicken breasts with 1 teaspoon of the olive oil and season them with ½ teaspoon of the salt, ¼ teaspoon of the pepper, and the turmeric. Place the chicken on the pan.

In a medium bowl, combine the zucchini, squash, onion, and tomatoes. Add the parsley and oregano and then drizzle with the remaining 1 tablespoon olive oil. Toss the vegetables well until they are evenly coated, and spread around the chicken breasts on the pan.

Bake in the center of the oven for 15 minutes, turn over the chicken and stir the vegetables, and then bake for 10 to 12 minutes more, or until the chicken juices run clear.

To serve, place 1 breast on each plate and top with one-quarter of the vegetables.

Yields 4 servings.

Easy Chicken Pasta Soup

Boil the pasta a day or two ahead of time and after draining, place it in a resealable bag in the fridge until ready to use. This bit of prep work makes this soup a lunch that takes just ten minutes to make.

- 3 cups chicken stock
- 1 cup frozen green beans
- 1 cup frozen sliced carrots
- 1 (6-ounce) can flaked chicken, drained
- 1 teaspoon chopped fresh tarragon
- 1 teaspoon fresh thyme leaves
- ½ teaspoon salt
- ¼ teaspoon freshly ground black pepper
- 1 cup cooked mini-shell pasta
- ½ cup shredded Parmesan cheese

In a large saucepan, bring the chicken stock to a boil over high heat. Add the green beans and carrots, and reduce the heat to medium. Cover and let simmer for 5 minutes.

Add the chicken, tarragon, thyme, salt, and pepper, and simmer for 4 minutes more.

Remove the pan from the heat and stir in the cooked pasta.

To serve, divide between 4 bowls and top with the Parmesan.

Yields 4 servings.

Seafood-Stuffed Avocadoes

This is a great light lunch, especially during the warmer months. You can prepare the filling up to three days ahead and just assemble the dish when you're ready to eat.

- 1 cup cooked cocktail shrimp
- 8 ounces imitation flaked crabmeat, chopped
- 1 stalk celery, finely chopped
- ½ red bell pepper, chopped
- ½ red onion, chopped
- 2 scallions, sliced
- 2 tablespoons light mayonnaise
- 1 tablespoon plain yogurt
- ¼ teaspoon dry mustard
- 2 tablespoons chopped fresh parsley
- ½ teaspoon freshly ground black pepper
- 2 avocados
- 1 teaspoon lemon juice

In a medium mixing bowl, combine the shrimp, crabmeat, celery, bell pepper, onion, and scallions; mix well.

In a small bowl, combine the mayonnaise, yogurt, dry mustard, parsley, and black pepper, and stir with a fork until well combined.

Combine the mayonnaise mixture with the seafood filling until well blended.

Cut the avocados in half, remove the pits, and wipe the flesh with the lemon juice.

Fill each avocado half with one-quarter of the seafood filling and serve.

Yields 4 servings.

Chopped BLT Salad

This salad lets you enjoy all the flavors of the classic BLT sandwich without going overboard on fat and calories. Using turkey bacon and croutons (instead of bread) go a long way toward making this a healthier way to have a BLT.

- 4 slices turkey bacon
- 2 cups chopped iceberg lettuce
- 2 medium tomatoes, diced
- ½ cup plain croutons
- 1 tablespoon mayonnaise
- 1 tablespoon light Italian dressing

Prepare the turkey bacon in the microwave according to package directions. Allow it to drain on paper towels and cool for 5 minutes.

Meanwhile, combine the lettuce, tomatoes, and croutons in a large bowl.

In a small cup, stir together the mayonnaise and Italian dressing (it will be thick).

Crumble the bacon and add to the salad. Pour the dressing over all and stir well until the salad is well coated. Divide between 2 plates and serve.

Yields 2 servings.

Power-Packed Green Smoothie

Even if you don't have time for much of a lunch, you'll still have time to get a heaping helping of vitamins and minerals in the form of this smoothie. The healthy fat from the avocado and the fiber from the vegetables mean you'll feel satisfied, too.

- 1 medium cucumber, peeled and chopped
- 2 cups fresh baby spinach
- ½ cup fresh parsley
- 1 cup carrot juice
- ½ teaspoon salt
- 2 dashes red pepper hot sauce
- ½ avocado, chopped

Combine the cucumber, spinach, parsley, carrot juice, salt, and hot sauce in a blender and blend on high until smooth.

Add the avocado and blend on medium speed until smooth. Divide between 4 glasses and serve immediately.

Yields 4 servings.

Toasted Ham, Swiss, and Arugula Sandwiches

This toasted sandwich omits the fat of the typical grilled ham and cheese and adds a lot more crunch. Served with a light soup or a salad, this is a delicious and healthy lunchtime meal.

- 8 slices reduced-calorie whole wheat bread
- 2 teaspoons Dijon mustard
- 1 pound (about 16 slices) thinly sliced lean deli ham
- 8 slices reduced-fat Swiss cheese
- 1 cup fresh arugula

Preheat the oven to 350 degrees F.

Spread 4 slices of the bread with the Dijon mustard, and top with about 4 slices of ham and 2 slices of cheese.

Top each with ¼ cup arugula and place the remaining bread slices onto the sandwiches. Bake in the center of the oven for 5 minutes, turn over, and then bake for 3 minutes more, or until the bread is golden and the cheese is melted. Cut each sandwich in half and serve hot.

Yields 4 servings.

Quick and Light White Bean Chili

This chili takes no time (and only one pan) to cook, and it tastes even better the next day. It also freezes well, so make a double batch to portion and store in the freezer for busy days.

- 1 teaspoon olive oil
- 1 pound freshly ground turkey breast
- 1 teaspoon chili powder
- 1 teaspoon salt
- ½ teaspoon freshly ground black pepper
- ½ teaspoon ground cumin
- 1 cup diced white onion
- 2 tablespoons chopped fresh cilantro
- 2 (15-ounce) cans great northern beans, undrained
- 2 cups chicken stock

In a medium heavy saucepan, heat the olive oil over medium-high heat. Add the turkey, chili powder, salt, pepper, and cumin and sauté and saute for 7 to 8 minutes, chopping often with the spatula, until the turkey is cooked through.

Add the onion and sauté for 1 minute more before adding the cilantro, beans with liquid, and chicken stock. Bring to a boil, then reduce the heat to low, cover, and let simmer for 15 minutes. Divide between 4 soup bowls and serve hot.

Yields 4 servings.

Vegetable Market Scramble

There's nothing wrong with breakfast for lunch. This dish cooks up in just a few minutes and will keep you going all day long.

- 1 teaspoon olive oil
- ½ red bell pepper, diced
- ½ cup diced white onion
- 1 cup sliced fresh mushrooms
- ½ teaspoon salt
- ¼ teaspoon freshly ground black pepper
- 8 large eggs, beaten

In a large heavy skillet, heat the olive oil over medium heat. Add the bell pepper, onion, mushrooms, salt, and pepper and sauté for 5 minutes, stirring frequently.

Pour the eggs over all and scramble, stirring constantly, for about 3 minutes, or until the eggs are set. Divide between 4 plates and serve hot.

Yields 4 servings.

Eggplant, Hummus, and Goat Cheese Sandwiches

Grilled slices of eggplant replace deli meats, and hummus adds protein and fiber while taking the place of mayonnaise. Try this classic Greek recipe and bring a Mediterranean flair to your lunch table.

- 1 medium eggplant, sliced ½ inch thick
- Sea salt
- 2 tablespoons olive oil
- Freshly ground black pepper
- 5 to 6 tablespoons hummus
- 4 slices whole wheat bread, toasted
- 1 cup baby spinach leaves
- 2 ounces goat cheese or feta cheese, softened

Preheat a gas or charcoal grill to medium-high heat.

Salt both sides of the sliced eggplant, and let it sit for 20 minutes to draw out the bitter juices.

Rinse the eggplant and pat dry with a paper towel.

Brush the eggplant with the olive oil and season to taste with salt and pepper.

Grill the eggplant until lightly charred on both sides but still slightly firm in the middle, 3 to 4 minutes per side.

Spread the hummus on 2 slices of the bread and top with the spinach leaves, goat cheese, and eggplant. Top with the remaining slices of bread and serve warm.

Yields 2 servings.

HEALTHY RECIPES FOR NON-FASTING DAYS: DINNER

> **Note on Non-Fasting Day Recipes:** The recipes for non-fasting days are low in calories but suitable for guests or the entire family, so we've created most of them to make four servings. If you like, you can either halve the ingredients or freeze extra servings for easy reheating on another day.

Tangy Orange Chicken Breast

This recipe delivers on both speed and flavor. It's a terrific dish to whip up on busy nights. Served with a green salad and some quinoa or brown rice, it's a light but satisfying meal.

- 1 teaspoon olive oil
- 4 (4- to 5-ounce) skinless chicken breasts
- 1 teaspoon paprika
- ½ teaspoon salt
- ¼ teaspoon freshly ground black pepper
- 1 teaspoon chopped fresh thyme
- 1 teaspoon chopped fresh rosemary
- 1 tablespoon unsweetened orange juice concentrate
- 2 tablespoons chopped fresh parsley

Preheat the oven to 400 degrees F and line a baking dish with aluminum foil. Spread the olive oil all over the bottom of the dish.

Place the chicken breasts in the dish, flip over to coat with oil, and season with the paprika, salt, pepper, thyme, and rosemary.

Bake for 15 minutes, then flip the chicken and brush with the orange juice concentrate. Bake for 15 to 20 minutes more, or until the chicken juices run clear.

Garnish with the parsley before serving.

Yields 4 servings.

Grilled Shrimp and Black Bean Salad

This recipe is a great one to use when you have company for dinner. No one will think it's low calorie!

- 1 teaspoon lime zest (about ½ lime)
- ¼ cup freshly squeezed lime juice
- 3 tablespoons olive oil
- 2 tablespoons chopped fresh basil
- 2 tablespoons chopped fresh oregano
- 1 teaspoon freshly ground black pepper
- ½ teaspoon salt
- 2 (15-ounce) cans black beans, rinsed and drained
- 1 cup diced tomatoes
- 1 cup diced green bell pepper
- ½ cup chopped green onions
- 24 large (21–25 count) raw shrimp, peeled and deveined

In a medium bowl, combine the lime zest and juice, olive oil, basil, oregano, and pepper and mix well. Measure 2 tablespoons out into a small bowl and set aside.

Add the salt, black beans, tomatoes, bell pepper, and onions to the medium bowl and toss well. Place in the refrigerator until serving.

Preheat a flat grill over medium-high heat. Once hot, place the shrimp on the grill and baste with the reserved lime juice mixture. Cook for 3 minutes on one side and then turn, baste again, and cook for 3 minutes more.

To serve, place one-quarter of the bean salad onto each plate and top with 6 hot shrimp.

Yields 4 servings.

Mustard-Maple-Glazed Salmon

This is an incredibly delicious recipe for salmon, especially given how quick and simple it is to prepare. Add a baked sweet potato or some brown rice and you have a flavorful, rich meal.

- 4 (6-ounce) skin-on salmon fillets, ¾ inch thick
- 1 teaspoon olive oil
- ½ teaspoon salt
- ½ teaspoon freshly ground black pepper
- 2 tablespoons pure maple syrup
- ½ teaspoon dry mustard
- 8 sprigs fresh thyme

Preheat a flat grill over medium-high heat.

Brush the salmon fillets on both sides with the olive oil, season with salt and pepper, and place them skin side down on the grill. Cook for 7 minutes.

Meanwhile, combine the maple syrup and dry mustard with a fork.

Flip the salmon fillets, brush with the maple-mustard glaze, and top each one with 2 sprigs of the thyme. Grill for 5 to 7 minutes more, or until the fish flakes easily.

To serve, use a spatula to transfer the fillets to 4 plates, leaving the thyme intact.

Yields 4 servings.

Tuscan-Style Baked Sea Bass

Sea bass is a tasty fish—fine and flaky. This Tuscan-inspired recipe complements this mild fish with the flavors of fresh tomatoes, walnuts, basil, and garlic.

- 4 (6-ounce) skin-on sea bass fillets
- 1 teaspoon olive oil
- 1 cup very finely chopped walnuts (use processor or blender)
- 2 teaspoons minced garlic
- 8 slices yellow or orange tomatoes, ¼ inch thick
- 8 slices red onion, ¼ inch thick
- ½ cup chopped fresh basil
- ½ teaspoon salt
- ¼ teaspoon freshly ground black pepper

Preheat the oven to 400 degrees F and line a baking sheet with aluminum foil.

Brush both sides of the bass fillets with the olive oil and then dip in the chopped walnuts, covering the fillets fully. Place the fillets skin side down on the baking sheet. Spread the garlic over the fillets, then cover the fish with alternating tomato and onion slices. Sprinkle the basil over the top and season with salt and pepper.

Bake for 12 to 14 minutes, or until the fish flakes easily.

To serve, use a spatula to transfer the fillets to 4 plates.

Yields 4 servings.

Portobello Cheeseburgers

You don't have to be a vegetarian to love these burgers, made with succulent portobello mushrooms. They're deliciously different but every bit as satisfying as a traditional burger, without all the fat and calories. Cannellini beans tucked under the caps make them filling enough for even the hungriest eater.

- 4 large (4 inches wide) portobello mushroom caps
- 1½ teaspoons olive oil, divided
- ½ teaspoon salt
- ¼ teaspoon freshly ground black pepper
- ½ teaspoon minced garlic
- ½ teaspoon paprika
- 1 cup canned cannellini beans
- 4 (1-ounce) slices reduced-fat mozzarella cheese
- 4 whole wheat hamburger buns
- 4 large leaves romaine lettuce
- 4 slices fresh tomato
- 8 slices red onion

Preheat the oven to 325 degrees F.

Rub the cap sides of the mushrooms with ½ teaspoon of the olive oil and season with salt and pepper.

In a large skillet, heat the remaining 1 teaspoon olive oil over medium-high heat. Add the mushrooms, cap side down, and sauté for 4 minutes.

Meanwhile, mix together the garlic, paprika, and beans and heat in the microwave for 1 minute, or just until warm. Set aside.

Flip the mushrooms and place 1 slice of mozzarella onto each one. Reduce the heat to low.

Toast the hamburger buns in the oven for 5 minutes, or just until crisp. Transfer to 4 plates. Top the bottom buns with the lettuce, tomato, and onion.

Spoon one-quarter of the bean mixture into a mound in the center of each bun and top with a mushroom, cap side up. Add the top buns and serve.

Yields 4 servings.

Flank Steak Spinach Salad

Flank steak is a lean and flavorful cut of meat that is ideal for a low-calorie diet. This recipe calls for the steak to be cooked medium rare. The meat tends to get quite tough if cooked much more than that.

- 1 pound flank steak, visible fat and sinew removed
- ¼ cup Balsamic Vinaigrette (see Avocado and Fennel Salad with Balsamic Vinaigrette recipe for directions), divided
- ½ teaspoon salt
- ½ teaspoon freshly ground black pepper
- 3 cups chopped romaine lettuce
- 1 cup baby spinach leaves
- 1 pint cherry tomatoes, halved
- ½ cup thinly sliced sweet yellow onion

Preheat a flat grill over high heat until it is very hot.

Brush the flank steak with 2 tablespoons of the Balsamic Vinaigrette, season with the salt and pepper, and place on the grill. Cook for 5 minutes, then flip and cook for 10 minutes more, or until the steak is medium rare.

Meanwhile, combine the lettuce, spinach, tomatoes, and onion until well mixed. Then add the remaining 2 tablespoons vinaigrette dressing. Toss well to coat and divide the salad between 4 plates.

Transfer the flank steak to a plate and allow it to rest for 10 minutes before slicing thinly on the diagonal.

Place one-quarter of the sliced steak on top of each salad and serve.

Yields 4 servings.

Chicken Picadillo

This variation on a traditional Latin dish uses leaner chicken in place of beef. It takes nothing away from the zesty flavor, but it does reduce the fat and calories usually present in the traditional version. Make an extra batch to freeze for later.

- 2 teaspoons olive oil
- ½ cup chopped yellow onion
- 2 cloves garlic, chopped
- ½ pound ground chicken
- ½ teaspoon ground cumin
- ½ teaspoon salt
- ¼ teaspoon freshly ground black pepper
- 2 tablespoons red wine
- 1 cup chopped tomato
- 1 fresh jalapeño pepper, seeded and diced
- ¼ cup green olives with pimientos, chopped
- 1 teaspoon Worcestershire sauce
- ¼ cup chopped fresh cilantro
- 1 teaspoon fresh lime juice (about ½ lime)

In a large heavy skillet, heat the olive oil over medium-high heat. Add the onion and garlic and sauté for 2 minutes, stirring often.

Add the chicken, cumin, salt, and pepper and cook for 5 to 6 minutes, stirring frequently to crumble the chicken.

Add the wine to the pan to deglaze it, scraping any browned bits from the bottom. Add the tomato, jalapeño, olives, and Worcestershire sauce; reduce the heat to medium and let simmer for 6 to 8 minutes, or until the mixture has thickened.

To serve, ladle into 4 bowls and finish with a squeeze of lime and a sprinkling of cilantro.

Yields 4 servings.

Chicken Florentine-Style

In this riff on true Florentine dishes, chicken breasts are treated with a delicious creamy sauce studded with fresh spinach. Serve this one to your guests—they'll have no idea you're on a diet.

- 1 teaspoon olive oil
- 4 (6-ounce) boneless skinless chicken breasts
- ½ teaspoon salt
- ¼ teaspoon freshly ground black pepper
- ¼ cup dry white wine
- ¼ cup chopped yellow onion
- 1 cup sliced fresh mushrooms
- 1 cup frozen chopped spinach, thawed and drained
- ½ cup chicken stock
- ¼ cup low-fat milk
- ¼ cup shredded Parmesan cheese

In a large heavy skillet, heat the olive oil over medium-high heat.

Season the chicken breasts on both sides with the salt and pepper and sauté for 5 minutes. Flip the chicken and cook for 5 to 7 minutes more, or until the juices run clear. Transfer to a plate and cover to keep warm.

Add the wine to the pan to deglaze it, and scrape up any browned bits from the bottom.

Add the onion, mushrooms, spinach, and chicken stock, and simmer for 10 to 15 minutes, or until the sauce is reduced by half.

Reduce the heat to medium, stir in the milk, and heat just until warmed though, about 1 minute.

To serve, place 1 chicken breast on each plate, top with one-quarter of the sauce, and sprinkle with the Parmesan cheese.

Yields 4 servings.

Easy Black Bean Soup

When served with a fresh salad and a crusty roll, this dish is a comforting and filling meal. You'll get all the flavors of traditional black bean soup but in far less time.

- 2 (15-ounce) cans black beans
- 2 cups chicken stock
- 1 cup thinly sliced carrots
- ½ cup chopped yellow onion
- ½ teaspoon garlic powder
- ½ teaspoon ground cumin
- ½ teaspoon chili powder
- ½ teaspoon salt
- ¼ teaspoon freshly ground black pepper
- 1 cup plain yogurt
- ¼ cup sliced green onions

In a large saucepan over medium-high heat, combine the black beans, chicken stock, carrots, onion, garlic powder, cumin, chili powder, and salt. Stir well.

Bring the soup to a boil, reduce the heat to medium, cover, and simmer for 20 minutes, stirring occasionally.

To serve, ladle into 4 bowls, top with a large dollop of yogurt, and garnish with green onions.

Yields 4 servings.

Hearty Vegetable Soup

This soup is easy to make and is just packed with a wide variety of vegetables. It's a great soup to serve alongside a salad or sandwich on those nights when you don't feel like cooking, so double up and freeze the extra.

- 1 teaspoon olive oil
- 1 cup diced Yukon Gold potatoes
- ½ cup thinly sliced carrots
- ½ cup fresh green beans, cut into 1-inch pieces
- ½ cup chopped yellow onion
- 1 cup fresh spinach leaves
- 3 cups chicken stock
- ¼ cup chopped fresh parsley
- 1 tablespoon chopped fresh rosemary
- ½ teaspoon salt
- ¼ teaspoon freshly ground black pepper

In a large heavy skillet, heat the olive oil over medium-high heat. Add the potatoes, carrots, green beans, and onion and sauté for 5 minutes, stirring frequently. Remove from the heat.

Transfer the vegetables to a large saucepan over medium-high heat. Add the spinach, chicken stock, parsley, rosemary, salt, and pepper and bring the soup to a boil. Reduce the heat to medium, cover, and simmer for 30 minutes.

To serve, ladle into 4 bowls.

Yields 4 servings.

Mushroom-Stuffed Zucchini

Fresh zucchini and mushrooms seasoned with garlic, olive oil, parsley, and Italian herbs and spices hardly seems like diet food. These mushroom-stuffed zucchini boats make an easy and impressive dish that is low in calories but still plenty filling. Serve with a piece of fish for dinner, or serve alone for lunch.

- 2 tablespoons olive oil
- 2 cups finely chopped button mushrooms
- 2 cloves garlic, finely chopped
- 2 tablespoons chicken stock
- 1 tablespoon finely chopped flat-leaf parsley
- 1 tablespoon Italian seasoning
- Sea salt
- Freshly ground black pepper
- 2 medium zucchini, cut in half lengthwise
- 1 tablespoon water

Preheat the oven to 350 degrees F.

Heat a large skillet over medium heat, and add the olive oil. Add the mushrooms and cook until tender, about 4 minutes. Add the garlic and cook for 2 minutes more. Add the chicken stock and cook for 3 to 4 minutes more.

Add the parsley and Italian seasoning, then season with salt and pepper to taste. Stir well and remove from the heat.

Scoop out the seeds and some of the flesh of the halved zucchini and stuff the halves with the mushroom mixture.

Place the zucchini in a casserole dish, and drizzle 1 tablespoon water in the bottom.

Cover with aluminum foil and bake for 30 to 40 minutes, or until the zucchini boats are tender.

Transfer to 2 plates and serve immediately.

Yields 2 servings.

Zesty Beef Kabobs

Tender, juicy, and zesty, these kabobs are going to make you glad you're eating healthy. Yet more proof that eating lean doesn't have to taste unappetizing!

- ½ cup lime juice
- 1 teaspoon salt
- 1 teaspoon black pepper
- 1 clove garlic, minced
- ¼ teaspoon red pepper flakes
- ¼ teaspoon rosemary, chopped
- ¼ teaspoon basil, chopped

- 1 pound lean red meat, such as beef, venison, or bison, chunked into bite-sized cubes
- 1 red onion, peeled, cut in half horizontally, and quartered vertically
- 1 pack cherry tomatoes
- 2 green peppers, cut similarly to the onion

Mix together the first seven ingredients.

Add meat to a large plastic zip bag, and pour the lime and spice mixture over it. Marinate for at least 20 minutes—the longer the better.

Preheat grill to medium/high when you're ready to make the kabobs.

Thread the meat, onions, tomatoes, and peppers onto your skewers.

Grill 1–3 minutes on each of the four sides, or until your steak reaches desired temp.

Yields 4 servings.

LOW-CALORIE DESSERT AND TREAT OPTIONS

Everyone likes a little something sweet now and then, especially when they've been behaving well on a low-calorie diet. Fruits are always a great sweet treat, and for those times when you'd like something a little more special, we've added some choices that can be had for 100 calories or less.

Feel free to indulge when you have a craving, but make sure that you're limiting these treats to just once a day or rewarding yourself even more occasionally. It's still important to try to keep sugar intake to a minimum, even on non-fasting days, so that your body's insulin and glucose levels begin to reach a healthier, more balanced state.

Apple juice or cider, ½ cup	60	calories
Blueberries, 1 cup	85	calories
Caramels, 2 pieces	80	calories
Cherries, ¼ cup dried	100	calories
Chocolate milk, ½ cup fat free	75	calories
Chocolate pudding, 1 fat-free (4-ounce) container	60	calories
Chocolate sandwich cookies, 2	100	calories
Dark chocolate, 1 ounce	100	calories
Figs, 2	80	calories
Fruit yogurt, ½ cup fat-free blended	90	calories

Frozen yogurt, ½ cup fat free	95	calories
Jelly beans, 20 small	90	calories
Kiwis, 2 medium	95	calories
Oatmeal cookies, 2 small	100	calories
Pineapple, 1 cup fresh	75	calories
Pomegranate juice, ⅔ cup	90	calories
Prune juice, ½ cup	90	calories
Strawberry sorbet, 1 small scoop	100	calories
Vanilla low-fat frozen yogurt, 1 small scoop	90	calories
Watermelon, 2 cups	90	calories

CONCLUSION

Making any healthy lifestyle change requires some determination and commitment. Adjusting to a healthy diet of whole foods can be daunting, especially if you've been eating a typical Western diet full of convenience foods, fast food, and sugar-laden treats.

However, the change in your body, your energy levels, and the way you feel about yourself after a few weeks on the 5:2 Fast Diet will make all of your hard work very worthwhile. Many people report that they feel much more energized and focused after just a week or two. If your goal is to lose excess weight and body fat, you'll likely see results within the first week.

More importantly, the changes you make to your diet, accompanied by regular exercise, will do so much more than make you feel better and look slimmer. They'll contribute to your overall health and can help prevent so many of the nutrition-related diseases and conditions that we see today.

While looking great is its own reward, the importance of making a positive impact on the length and quality of your life can't be overstated.

So when you feel tempted by old eating habits or the occasional craving, grab a healthy snack and reread the tips on motivation that we've provided, go for a long walk, or invite a friend to join you for one of your scheduled treats. Remembering why you're doing what you're doing and celebrating the way you look and feel can give you that boost you need to get over any bumps on the road to better health.

GLOSSARY

Blood sugar – the amount of glucose circulating through the bloodstream. Excess glucose that remains in the bloodstream (rather than being absorbed by the cells that need it) is often due to high sugar intake or insulin resistance.

Full fasting – going without food completely or eating very little food for prolonged periods, often five to ten days.

High-intensity interval training (HIIT) – intense cardio workouts alternating short bursts of intense physical activity with longer periods of moderate exercise. Workouts can be as short as seven minutes but typically last about twenty minutes.

Insulin – a hormone produced by the body that is responsible for transporting glucose through the phospholipid layer of the cells to be used as energy.

Insulin resistance – the lack of response to insulin by the body's cells. Often caused by excess abdominal and visceral fat and poor eating habits. Considered one of the markers of metabolic syndrome.

Intermittent fasting – fasting on alternate days, for certain hours during the day, or for very short periods.

Metabolic syndrome – a group of symptoms and conditions—including excess abdominal or visceral fat, insulin resistance, and hypertension—considered to be a precursor to type 2 diabetes.

Resistance training – also known as strength training. Exercise using body weight, free weights such as dumbbells, or weight machines to build lean muscle. Also improves bone density and has been shown to have a significant impact on heart health, weight loss, and longevity.

Type 2 diabetes – form of diabetes developed due to poor diet, obesity, and lack of exercise. Usually treated by diet, exercise, and possibly insulin injections.